MRI LAYMAN'S TERMS: THE BASIC CONCEPTS OF MRI PHYSICS MADE EASY

LAWRENCE MCNAIR JR
M.P.H., R.T. (R) (MR) (CT)

2nd Edition

PREFACE

As a struggling student while taking courses in magnetic resonance imaging, I found it difficult to comprehend some of the major concepts of MRI and its techniques. This is one of the reasons why I decided to write this manual on the physics of MRI. I hope this book will help students by making the concepts of MRI simpler, easier, and enjoyable for those who are preparing to become MRI Technologists. Hopefully with this book, your experiences will be less stressful. Although MRI is changing on a daily basis, the fundamental principles of MRI physics remain unchanged. I think this book will give you a positive outlook and help ease your anxiety toward the concepts of MRI.

CONTENTS

CHAPTER 1

BASIC PRINICPLES AND TERMS OF MRI

The concepts of magnetic resonance imaging (MRI) can be hard to comprehend. In the first section of this manual, some of the basic principles and terms are explained. It is important the simple principles and terms are comprehended in order to understand the more complex concepts explained later in this book. As with every discovery in medicine or science, every idea started off with a fundamental principle. The fundamental principle behind MRI involves the concepts of magnetism and charged particles.

Magnetism

Magnetism is a fundamental property of all matter because all materials are magnetic to some degree. In relation to MRI, there are three types of magnetism: ferromagnetism, paramagnetism, and diamagnetism.

Ferromagnetism materials are easily magnetic and have a magnetic susceptibility greater than 1. Some of these materials include: iron, cobalt, and nickel.

Paramagnetism materials are weakly influenced by magnets and have a magnetic susceptibility less than 1. Platinum, oxygen, tungsten, manganese and gadolinium are examples of paramagnetic agents.

Diamagnetic materials have negative magnetic susceptibilities and are slightly repelled by a magnet. These items include mercury, sliver, copper, carbon, and hydrogen.

Atomic Structure and Motion within the Atom

The atom consists of three main parts: electron, proton, and neutron. The nucleus of an atom contains proton and neutrons. This grouping of protons and neutrons are called nucleons.

- Listed is a diagram showing an atom and the motion within the atom.

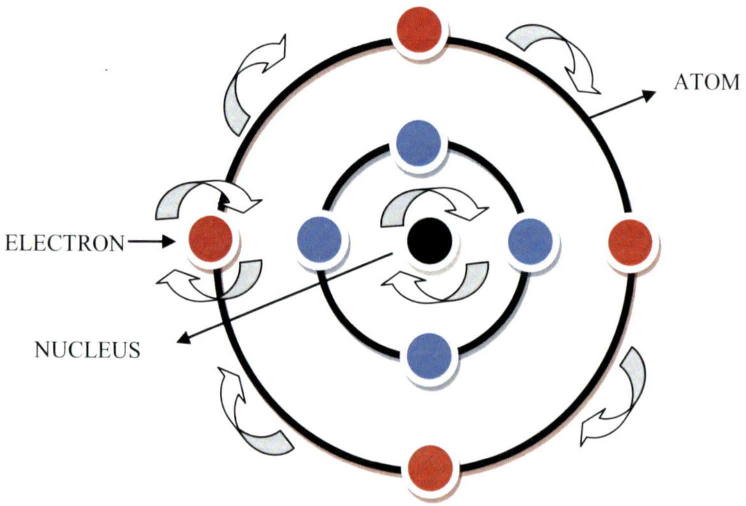

By looking at the diagram, there are three types of motion within an atom. There are:

1) The electron particles spinning on their own axis.

2) The electron particles orbiting the nucleus.

3) The nucleus spinning on its own cycle or axis.

Spin Quantum Number and Hydrogen (Most clinical isotope used in MRI)

Hydrogen atoms are the most clinically used because there are very abundant in the human body, 99% from water and fat. Hydrogen has an atomic and mass number of 1. Hydrogen also has a spin quantum number of ½ and a gyromagnetic ratio of 42.57 MHz/T or 42.6 MHz/T.

So what is a spin quantum number? A spin quantum number refers to the spin associated with a particle's nucleus. We learned in the last section, all particles are spinning continuously in space or around the nucleus of an atom. This spin induces the nuclear magnetic moment. For now, it is important to remember all particles have a spin quantum number (spin) associated with them. Another important thing to remember is this number determines rather a particle can be visualized with MRI or not. If the particle has a non-zero number, it can be visualized. If the particle has a zero number, it can't be visualized.

Some Layman's Terms

Before we go any further, let's introduce some Layman's terms that are important to become familiar with before we proceed.

- **Magnetic moment** (sometimes called net magnetization vector or bulk magnetization) - This is the vector left over once all of the other particles or protons have been canceled out. For example:

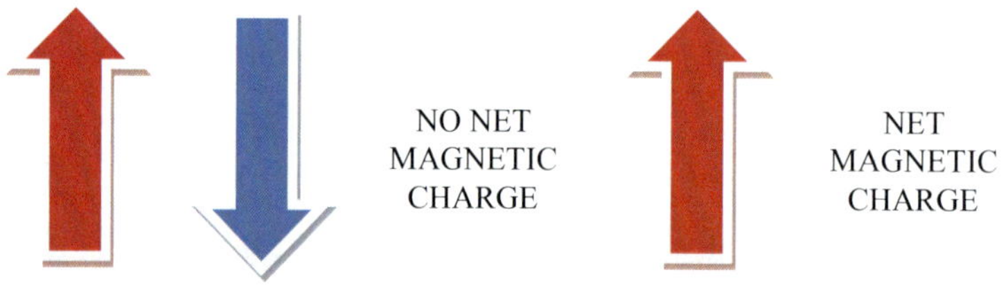

The magnetic moment has the properties of a vector, which means it has a size and a direction.

- **Static external magnetic field** (sometimes called B_o field) - This is another name for the magnet itself. This is saying the net magnetic moment is at rest.

- **Tesla** (T) – This is the unit of B_o or the magnet. For example, some magnets are 1.0 Tesla,1.5 Tesla, etc.

- **Gauss** (G) - This is the unit of the Tesla. For example, 1 Tesla = 10,000 Gauss

Alignment of Spins

Earlier we learned "all particles have a spin associated with them". This spin is the quantum spin number. We also learned "protons, located inside of the nucleus, spin on their own axis". With this being stated, protons in the environment as well as our bodies are spinning randomly.

The concept of alignment of spins says if randomly spinning protons are placed inside of a strong static magnetic field (B_o), the spins will align with or against the magnetic field. A magnet has a positive and negative pole. In MRI terms, it is called the higher energy state and the lower energy state. Some books refer to the higher energy state as anti parallel with the field and the lower energy state as parallel with the field. The terminology refers to the same concept.

Once the randomly spinning protons in our bodies are placed inside of the magnetic field, some will align parallel and anti parallel to B_o. Due to the law of averages, more protons will align parallel with the field than anti parallel with the field. For example at a 1.5 tesla magnet, for every 2 million protons, there are 9-18 more protons aligned parallel with the field than anti parallel with the field. Protons aligned with the field and protons aligned anti parallel with the field cancels each other out leaving behind a net magnetic moment, which is usually present in the low energy state. The net magnetic moment plays a role in producing the MRI signal. If the net magnetization increases, the signal is better.

- Listed are factors that influence rather a proton will align parallel or anti parallel with the magnetic field.

1) **The size of the magnet** - as magnet strength increases, more protons will align parallel with the field.

2) **The thermal energy of the nuclei** - the more energy nuclei have, nuclei are able to reach the higher energy state from the lower energy state. This allows more nuclei to align anti parallel with the magnet field rather than parallel with the magnet field.

- Listed are factors that will influence the net magnetization vector.

1) **The size of the magnet** - as magnet strength increases, net magnetization vector increases also.

2) **Gyromagnetic ratio** - as gyromagnetic ratio increases, net magnetization vector increases also.

3) **Spin quantum number** - as spin quantum number increases, net magnetization vector increases also.

4) **Temperature** - As temperature decreases (gets colder), net magnetization increases. This is why the temperature, in the room, is kept between 65 and 75 degrees with a relative humidity of 50 to 70 degrees.

5) **Total number of spins** - as total number of spins increases, the net magnetization increases also.

- Listed is a diagram of the process of a net magnetization vector (net magnetic moment).

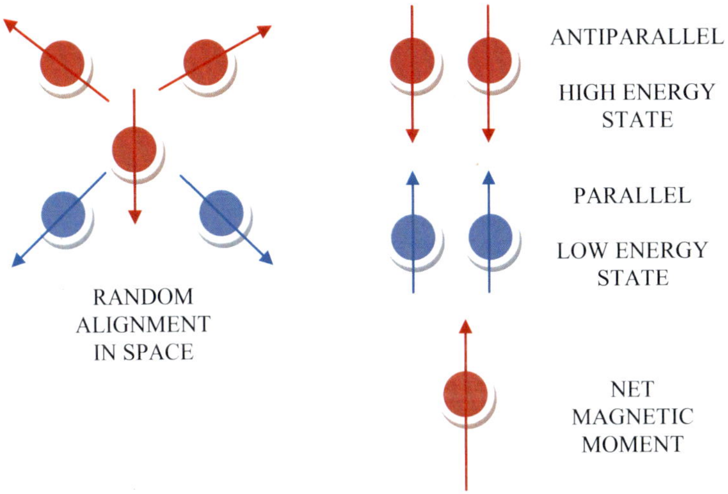

Precession and Larmor Equation

Protons of the hydrogen nucleus spin on their own axis. The concept of precession is the spinning of these protons once they are under the influence of the B_o field (magnet).

The secondary spinning that wobbles around the net magnetization vector of B_o is called precessional frequency. This frequency is measured in Megahertz (MHz) in which

1HZ is 1 cycle per second and 1 MHz is 1 million cycles per second.

The Larmor equation is an equation that measures the value of the precessional frequency. The formula for this equation is the:

$$\text{Precessional Frequency } (W_o) = B_o\, Y$$

- Where the B_o is the magnetic field strength of the magnet in (T).
- Where the Y is the gyromagnetic ratio in MHz / T

According to this equation, the bigger magnet strength and gyromagnetic ratio is, the faster the precession of a spin. For example for a hydrogen molecule at 1.5 T, the precessional frequency would be:

$$W_o = (1.5\ \text{T})\ (42.57) = 63.86\ \text{MHz}$$

Resonance

The topics up until this point have focused on the processing of spins at the B_o or stationary magnetic field level. Now let's discuss how molecules are moved from the longitudinal plane or z axis (B_o) to the transverse plane or x-y axis.

This movement deals with the term Resonance. Resonance is a phenomenon which occurs when an object is exposed to an oscillating perturbation that has a frequency close to its own natural frequency of oscillation. In layman's terms, the energy which comes from the radio pulse (RF) must equal the energy of the larmor frequency in order to move the molecule to the transverse plane or x-y plane (sometimes referred to as the B1 field). If the energy from the RF pulse does not equal the energy of the larmor frequency, of the particular molecule, it will not move.

The term that causes the RF pulse to bring a molecule into the state of resonance is called excitation. Excitation is another way of saying a molecule is excited by a particular RF pulse which will move it from the lower energy state to the higher energy state. Most of the time, a 90 degree RF pulse, called flip angle, is needed to move the molecule from the B_o field to the B1 field. Once the molecule or hydrogen is in the new B1 field, it will precess at the new level until relaxation occurs.

- Listed is a diagram of the principle of Resonance.

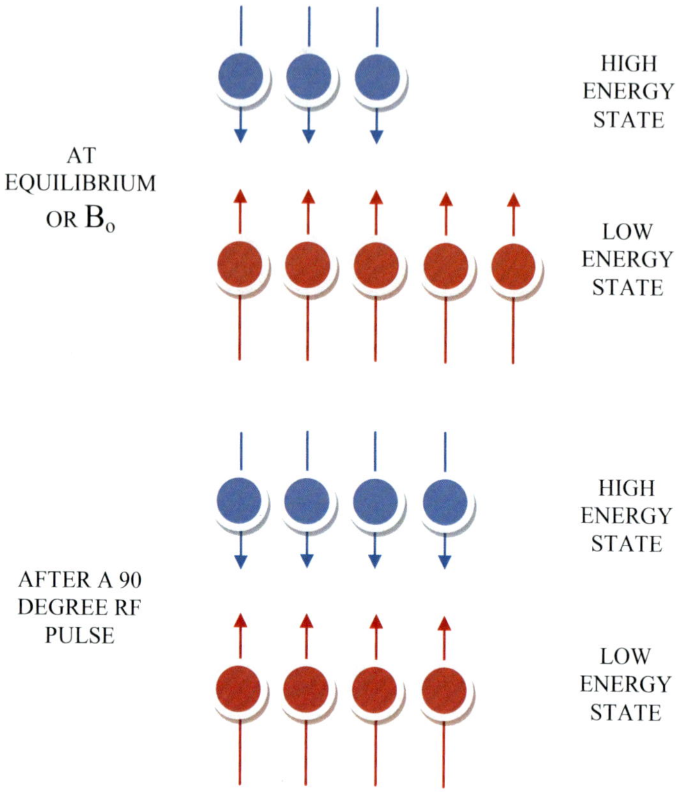

This new level the molecules are in refers to "in phase". This means the molecules are all symmetrical with each other.

Free Induction Decay Signal and Relaxation

In the last section, the concept of resonance was explained. Resonance caused the molecules, mainly hydrogen, to move from the B_0 field to the B1 field once the RF pulse is applied. This new level of placement was termed in phase.
The B_0 field tries to realign the in phase molecules, once the RF pulse are turned off. This process is called relaxation. There are two types of relaxation: T1 recovery and T2 decay.

T1 recovery is the rephasing of the longitudinal magnetization.

T2 decay is the dephasing of the transverse magnetization.

The signal collected from T1 recovery or the T2 decay is called the free induction decay or FID signal.

- When I first learned about Resonance, FID, and Relaxation, it was very confusing. One way to remember these concepts is to of think of them in relation to a toy yoyo. As a kid when you threw out a yoyo, it precesses in space. Then it tries to return to you. The same principle applies here. When a molecule is hit by a 90 degree RF pulse, it falls down 90 degrees but it always tries to return to its starting point. The time it takes the molecule to return back to equilibrium or Bo is the FID. The FID will be longitudinal or transverse magnetization depending on whether it is T1 recovery or T2 decay.

T1 Relaxation and T2 Relaxation

T1 relaxation is the time it takes to recover 63 % of the initial net magnetization. This refers to the longitudinal recovery of the FID. This relaxation is called spin- lattice. The concept is called spin lattice because as the net magnetization relaxes back to equilibrium, from a higher energy state to a lower energy state, energy is being given off to the environment (lattice) in order to do so.

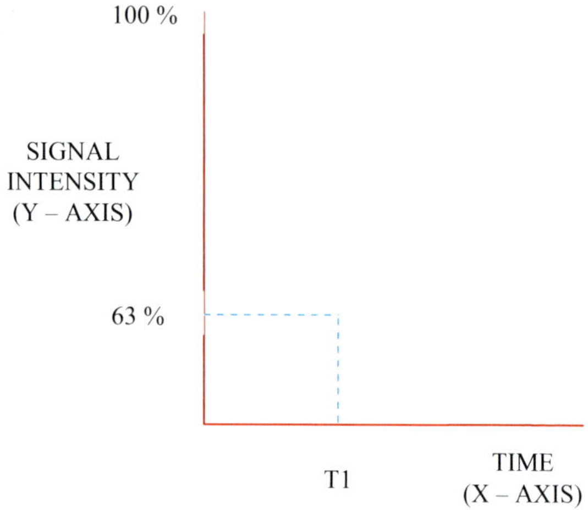

T2 relaxation, on the other hand, is the time it takes the net magnetization to lose 63 % of its signal. Since T2 relaxation involves a decaying process, it is designed to collect signal lost instead of signal gain. It is often called spin- spin because of the interactions between the magnetic fields of adjacent nuclei.

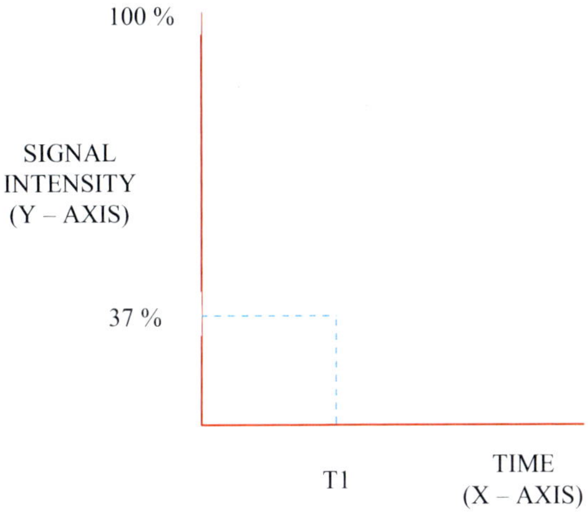

Repetition Time and Echo Time

Repetition Time (TR) is the time from the application of one RF pulse to the application of the next RF pulse. It is measured in milliseconds (ms or msec). TR also determines the amount of longitudinal relaxation which has occurred, making it the primary controller of T1 relaxation.
It is important to remember the TR stays on the whole time during the scan.

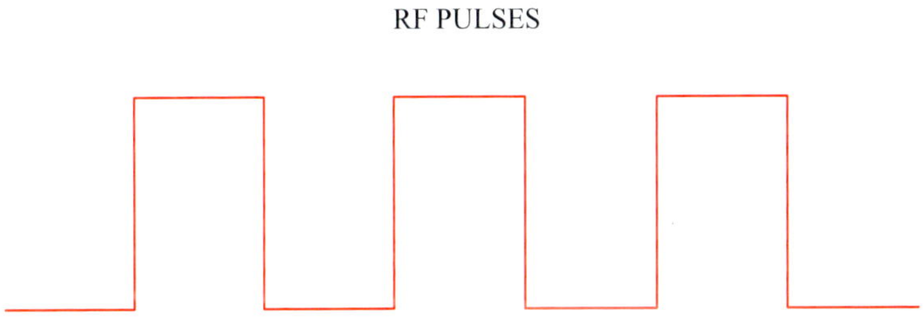

Echo Time (TE) is the time from the application of the RF pulse to the peak of the signal induced in the coil. TE is the primary controller of transverse magnetization decay, which is T2 relaxation.

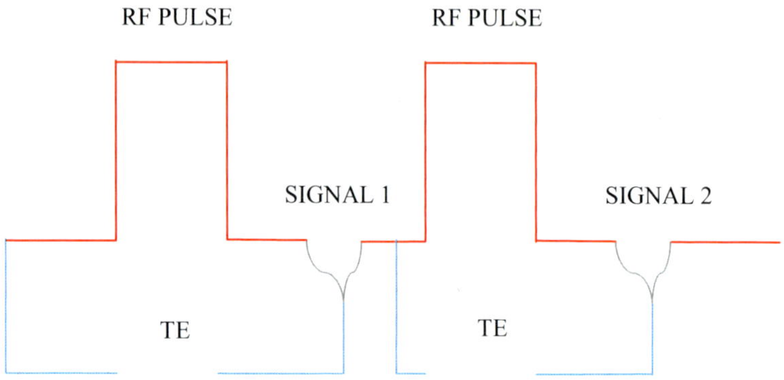

Faraday's Law of Induction

Before we move on to the next chapter, let's make sure the concept of Faraday's Law is comprehended. According to Faraday's Law, a moving magnetic field induces a voltage in a wire. This principle describes how MRI works. The changing magnetic field induces a voltage in a wire and the signal is collected.

Chapter 2

Contrast and Image Weighting

In MRI scanning, high resolution of contrast is the main reason MRI has the primary advantage over other modalities. Within this chapter, the differences between fat and water are explained. The concepts of image weighting for Spin Echo and Gradient Echo Sequences are also explained. The selections of imaging weighing parameters are explained as well. It is important the information, in this chapter, is comprehended. The usage of contrast and the selection of image weighting parameters are crucial when performing MRI scans.

What is Contrast?

In some modalities, contrast means the differences between shades of grays in an image. In MRI scanning, contrast means something different. It refers to "brightness" and "darkness". On a MRI scan, there will be areas of high density (light) and areas of low density (dark). Physicians or books may refer to these terms as hyperintense (light) or hypointense (dark). These terms are interchangeable.

In order to obtain these light and dark signals, the relaxation times of fat and water are manipulated. The FID also plays a role in our efforts to see the different between light and dark signals. The magnitude or size of the FID determines how bright or intense the MRI signal will be.

- Listed below is a way to remember this concept.

1. **Large FID = Bright Areas within an image**
2. **Small FID = Dark Areas Within an image**

Fat / Water

The concept of Fat verses water is an important principle involving MRI. Fat and water are the two most utilized compounds in MRI scanning because our bodies have an abundant supply. Fat and water has two different relaxation times. The relaxation time of fat is less than the relaxation time of water along the longitudinal axis. This means fat is able to recover quicker than water.

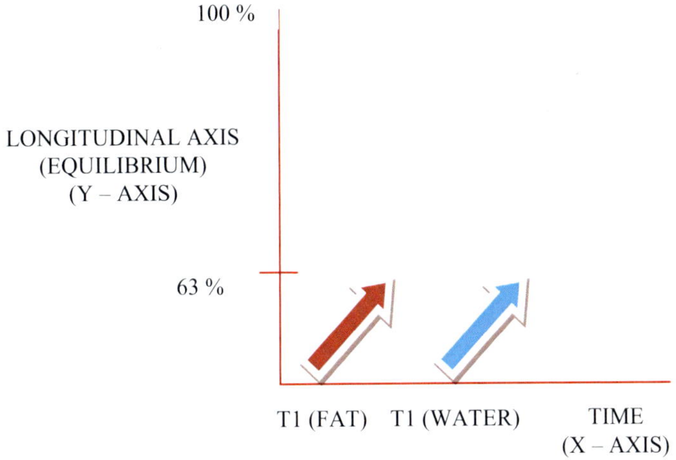

- Fat relaxation time is shorter than water causing it to recover quicker (T1).

The relaxation time of water is longer than the relaxation time of fat along the transverse axis. This means water requires a longer time to recover back to the transverse axis or equilibrium state.

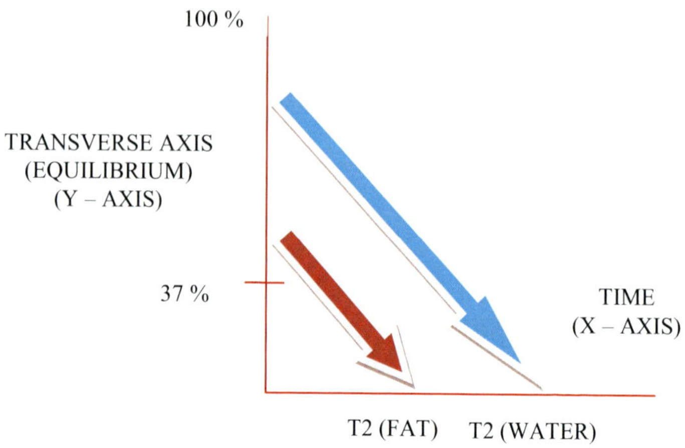

- Water relaxation time is longer than fat. It takes longer to recover.

T1 Contrast (Conventional Spin Echo)

T1 contrast utilizes the principle of fat verses water. In T1 weighting, the goal is to obtain a scan in which fatty substances in the body are bright and fluid substances are dark. This event happens due to the relaxation times between fat and water. T1 of fat is less than T1 of water; therefore, fat can recover quicker to the longitudinal axis. This allows the protons in fat to give off a bright FID (signal), which cause those areas to appear bright.

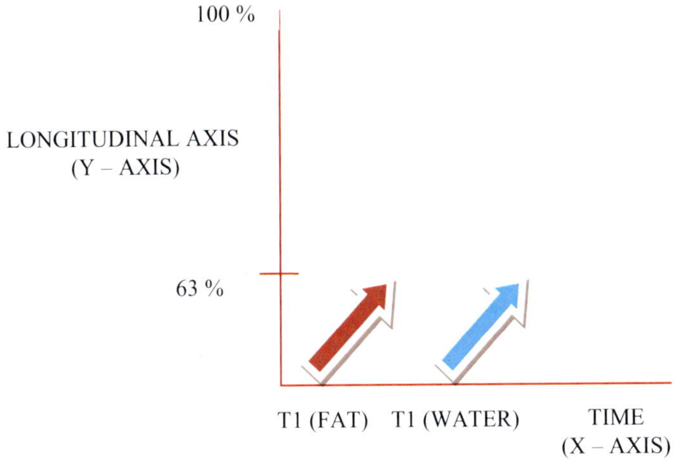

- Fat appears bright on a T1 weighted image while Water appears dark.

T2 Contrast (Conventional Spin Echo)

T2 contrast also utilizes the principle of fat verses water. In a T2 weighted image, the goal is to obtain an image in which fluid- filled substances appears bright and fatty substances appear dark. This event also happens due to the relaxation times between fat and water. T2 of water is longer than T2 of fat; therefore, water will take longer to decay to the transverse axis. This allows the protons in water to give off a bight FID (signal), which cause those areas to appear bright.

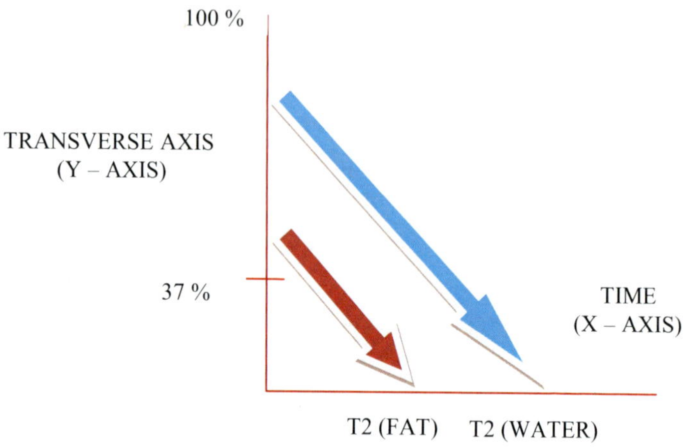

- Water appears bright on a T2 weighted image while Fat appears dark.

Proton Density Contrast (Conventional Spin Echo)

Proton Density (PD) utilizes the principle of protons within an area. In a PD weighted image, the areas with the most protons appears bright. The areas with the least amount of protons appear dark.

Usage of TR and TE in Image Weighting (Conventional Spin Echo)

The concepts of parameters and imaging weighting can be tough to comprehend. Let's explain them in layman's terms.

The usage of repetition time (TR) and echo time (TE) are the two main parameters used in imaging weighting. When examining contrast weighted images, the scan contrast you want to obtain must stand out from the contrast you do not want to obtain. In order to accomplish this for all three weighting (T1, T2, PD), the parameter which influences the scan should be dominant while the other parameter should be repressed.

For example, in a T1 weighted fatty substances need to be bright. Therefore, we must determine how the TR and TE times affect these. The relaxation time of fat is short and water relaxation time is long. Therefore the TR time, which is the primary controller of T1 relaxation, should be short in order to catch the effects of the fat before it has time to recover or relax back to the longitudinal axis.

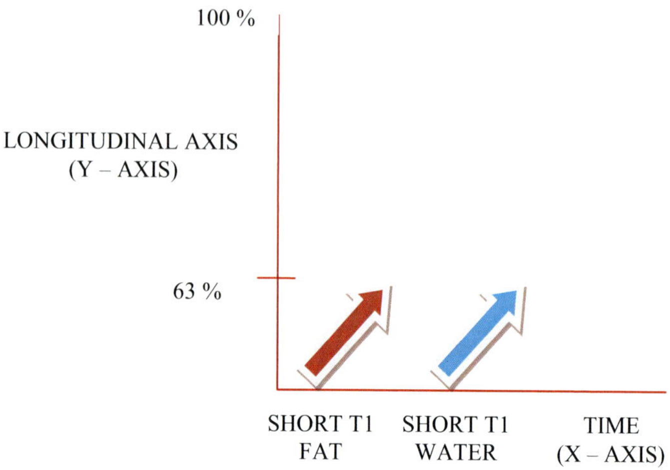

In a T2 weighted image, fluid- filled substances need to be bright. The TE time, which is the primary controller of T2 decay, should be long, in order to allow the effects of water to elapse. If the TE time is short, the effects will not have time to take place.

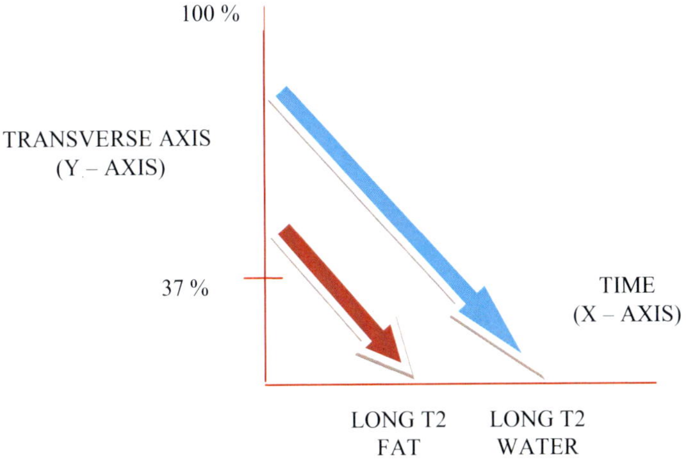

Summary of Image Weighting (Conventional Spin Echo)

The parameter which influences the scan is dominant while the other parameter is repressed. Applying this concept, there are two types of relaxation times: short and long.

- For a T1 weighted scan, if the TR time is short (dominant), the TE time is short in order to repress the decaying effect.

- For a T2 weighted scans, if the TE time is long (dominant) to allow the decaying effect, the TR time is long in order to repress the short T1 relaxation effect.

- For a PD weighted scan, this sequence depends on the presence of protons to be present. In order for the protons for the protons to be present, both the TR and the TE parameters are repressed. In this situation, the TR time is long in order to repress the short T1 relaxation effect. The TE time is short in order to repress the decaying effect.

Typical Values of TR and TE Times Used in MRI Scanning (Conventional Spin Echo)

Long TR	2000ms and above
Short TR	300ms – 950ms
Long TE	60ms and above
Short TE	10ms – 30ms

Contrast (Conventional Gradient Echo)

The usage of contrast in conventional gradient echo sequences is similar to the philosophy used in conventional spin echo sequences. Conventional gradient echo sequences still use the parameters TR and TE. The only difference is the usage of the flip angle parameter. The flip angle is an RF pulse, usually 90 degrees, which moves the molecule from the B_o field to the B1 field. In conventional gradient echo sequences, the flip angle can be between 5 – 110 degrees. The flip angle is the main parameter that affects contrast in conventional gradient echo sequences. Another important point to remember about conventional gradient echo sequences, in relation to contrast, is the TR time will always be short due to the speed of the scan.

T1 Weighted (Conventional Gradient Echo)

The principle is the same as conventional spin echo sequences. In order to see the desired effect of image weighting, the parameter must be dominant. In this case, it is the flip angle. A large flip angle is equivalent to a short TR time in conventional spin echo sequences. Therefore the TR time, for this particular image weighting, is short in order to maximize T1 effects and due to the speed of the scan. The TE time is also short in order to minimize the effects of T2*. The flip angle is large.

T2* Weighted (Conventional Gradient Echo)

In conventional gradient echo sequences, the value (T2*) takes the place of the value T2 used in conventional spin echo sequences. T2* is used due to the field imhomogeneities, loss of signal, of conventional gradient echo sequences. In order to see the desired effect of image weighting, the parameter must be dominant. In this case, it is the flip angle. A small flip angle (5 - 70 degrees) is equivalent to a long TR time in conventional spin echo sequences. The TR time, for this image weighting, is short instead of long due to the speed of the scan. The TE time is long in order to maximize T2* decay effects. The flip angle is small.

Proton Density Weighted (Conventional Gradient Echo)

This principle is also the same as conventional spin echo sequences. In order to obtain a PD weighted image, the TR time is short due to the speed of the scan. The TE time is short in order to minimize the effects of T2*. The flip angle is small.

Summary of Imaging Weighting (Conventional Gradient Echo)

The parameter which influences imaging weighting is dominant while the other parameters are repressed. Applying this concept, there are two relaxation times in conventional gradient echo sequences: short and long. The flip angles, small and large, determine the weighting of the image in this scan.

- For a T1 weighted image, the TR time is short to maximize T1 effects and due to the speed of the scan. The TE time is short in order to minimize T2* effects. The flip angle is large because it is the primary controller of T1 contrast in conventional gradient echo sequences.

- For a T2* weighted image, the TR time is short instead of long due to the speed of the scan. The TE time is long in order to maximize T2* effects. The flip angle is small because it is the primary controller of T2 * contrast in conventional gradient echo sequences.

- For a PD weighted scan, the TR time is short instead of long due to the speed of the scan. The TE time is short in order to minimize T2* effect. The flip is also short because it is the primary controller of PD contrast in conventional gradient echo sequences.

Typical Values of TR, TE, and Flip Angle (Conventional Gradient Echo Sequence)

Long TR	100ms and above
Short TR	less than 50ms
Short TE	5ms – 10ms
Large TE	15ms – 25ms
Small Flip Angle	5 – 70 degrees
Large Flip Angle	70 – 110 degrees

Chapter 3

Introduction to Conventional Spin Echo and the Conventional Gradient Echo Sequence

The Conventional Spin Echo and Conventional Gradient Echo Sequence are two of the most common sequences used in MRI. Although these sequences will be further explained in more detail later, let's introduce them before we move ahead. It is important to understand the concepts of these two sequences before we proceed to Spatial Localization and K – Space.

Conventional Spin Echo Sequence

Earlier in the book, the philosophy of magnetization relaxation was explained. Protons are randomly aligned in our bodies or space. Once these protons or spins are placed under the influence of a static magnetic field, some of them will align themselves parallel or anti parallel to B_o field. Following this event, the RF pulse is turned on and resonance occurs. The concept of resonance will force the spins, net magnetization, to move from the B_o field to the B1 field. Once the RF pulse is turned off, the spins will try to relax back to equilibrium. However, the spins are not refocused. Now let's look at the conventional spin echo sequence.

In conventional spin echo sequences, the net magnetization is forced out of the B_o field to the B1 field by the usage of a 90 degree flip angle or the optimal angle. Once this occurs, a second pulse is applied at 180 degree flip angle which refocuses the spins. The signal that occurs from the refocusing pulse or relaxation is called the free induction decay (FID) or echo. This process is called spin echo.

- Listed is a diagram for the Convention Spin Echo Sequence.

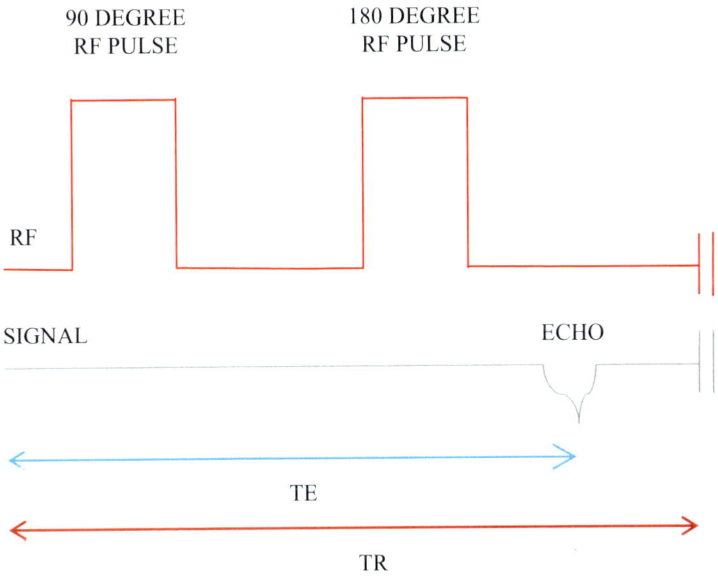

- This principle applies to whether the spin echo sequence is a single echo or multiple spin echo sequence. A double echo collects two signals, one for each echo.

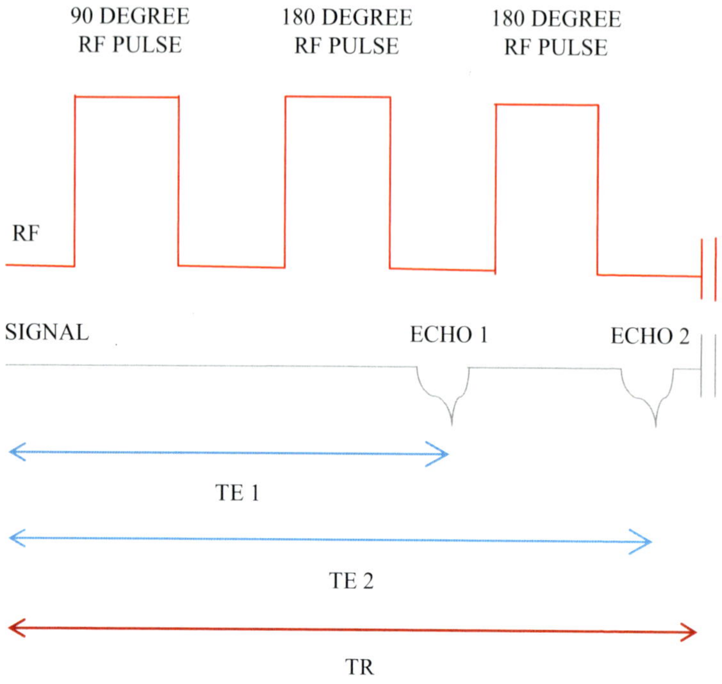

Conventional Gradient Echo Sequence

Conventional gradient echo sequences utilize the same philosophy as the conventional spin echo sequences. The only different between the two is the usage of a variable RF excitation pulse, flip angle, instead of a 90 degrees excitation pulse. Conventional gradient echo sequences also use a gradient reversal to refocus the spin, instead of the 180 degrees refocusing pulse used in the conventional spin echo sequences.

- Listed is a diagram for the Conventional Gradient Echo Sequence.

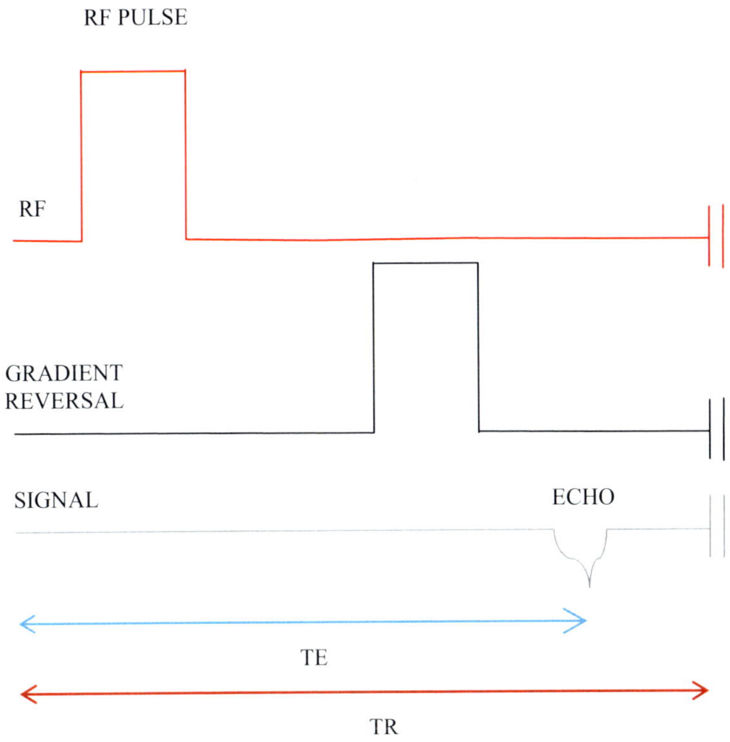

Chapter 4

Spatial Localization and K – Space

In MRI, Spatial Localization and K- Space are two important concepts. These principles deal with decoding the data and putting it into image form. In this chapter, the basics of each will be explained.

The Use of Gradients Magnetic Fields

Gradients are one of the most important terms that must be understood in order to perform MRI scans. MRI uses gradients in the majority of its functions. The main functions of gradients involve magnetization dephasing, refocusing and spatial localization.

So what is a gradient? Gradients are magnetic fields produced by running a current through the wires located inside of the magnet. In layman's terms, the magnetic field is created when the gradient super imposes itself over the static magnetic field or B_o. We learned in chapter one when spins are placed inside of the static magnetic field, they precess at a certain frequency. When these spins are encountered by the gradient magnetic field, they still precess at a certain frequency. However, the gradient magnetic field gives each spin a specific precessional frequency at a certain place inside of the magnet. This may be a little confusing. Let's put it in Layman's terms.

We know a magnet is not perfect. Although, a magnet has a magnetic strength of 1.0 Telsa, there are areas inside of the magnet that is not 1.0 telsa. For example, there may be an area of 0.5 or 0.8. The 1.0 Telsa represents the total weight of the magnet once each part within it is accounted for. This philosophy applies to the gradient magnetic field. When the gradient magnetic field is turned on, each spin inside of the body have a different precessional frequency. This difference in precessional frequency set the stage for spatial localization.

Spatial Localization (Slice Selection, Frequency Encoding, Phase Encoding)

Spatial Localization utilizes gradients. There are three gradient coils located inside of the magnet: x gradient, y gradient, and z gradient. The center point of these three gradients is called magnetic isocentre. The concept of spatial localization can be a tough one to comprehend. Let's discuss this process in layman's terms.

Slice Selection Gradient

When a body is placed inside of the magnetic field and the MRI scanner is turned on, a gradient is applied over the B_0 field. This gradient magnetic field gives the hydrogen spins a specific value at a certain place inside of the magnet. Once this occurs, a RF pulse is applied to the spins. During the TR period, the slice selection gradient is applied to the body, which will extract out a slab of tissue. The extraction of a certain tissue is carried out by applying resonance to the spins which have the same larmor frequency of the body part that you want to scan. For example, if you wanted to scan a right shoulder, only the spins in the shoulder will be excited.

The slice selection gradient also plays a role in the imaging plane you want to scan in. For example, of the three gradients (x, y, and z) if you want to scan in the axial plane, the z gradient will be selected. If you want to scan in the sagittal plane, the x gradient will be selected. If you want to scan in the coronal scan, the y gradient will be selected. After the imaging plane has been determined, a slice thickness is chosen. The gradient will either use a hard pulse or a soft pulse. A hard pulse is a strong B1 field RF pulse or a very large bandwidth of excitations. A soft pulse is a weak B1 field RF pulse or a very narrow bandwidth of excitations. Some books use the term "selective" for soft pulse or "non selective" for hard pulse. The formula for slice selection thickness is:

SS Thickness = Bandwidth of RF Excitation / Gradient Strength

- **This means to achieve more coverage on your slices, the RF transmit bandwidth will have to be increased or a shallow gradient slope must be used.**

- **To achieve less coverage on your slices, the RF transmit bandwidth will have to be decreased or a steep gradient slope must be used.**

Frequency Encoding Gradient

Once a slice undergoes slice selection, another gradient called frequency encoding is applied. The frequency encoding gradient or readout gradient collects the signals which come from the slice. The direction of the readout gradient is usually determined by the operator of the MRI machine. It is normally placed along the long axis of the anatomy in the frequency direction. This is done so all of the signals, rephasing and dephasing part of the echo as well as the peak, can be collected regardless of the size of the anatomy being scanned. The frequency encoding makes up one part of the field of view of the image.

Phase Encoding Gradient

Once the signals are obtained by the readout gradient in the frequency direction, the remaining signals are collected by the phase encoding gradient. The phase encoding gradient works by the gradient turning "on and off" at different times, during the scan, to catch the fast moving spins and slow moving spins. In conventional spin echo sequences, the gradient is usually turned on right before the 180 degrees refocusing pulse. In conventional gradient echo sequences, the gradient is turned on between the excitation of the spins and the collection of the echo. The phase encoding gradient is usually placed along the short axis of the anatomy, by the operator of the MRI machine. This is done to reduce scan time and to cut down on patient motion. The phase encoding gradient also makes up the other dimension of the field of view.

- Listed is a summary of which gradient are used in each imaging plane by the magnet.

	Sagittal	Axial (head)	Axial (body)	Coronal
SS	X	Z	Z	Y
PE	Y	X	Y	X
FE	Z	Y	X	Z

Sampling

Before we proceed to the principle of k– space, sampling is an important concept that needs to be explained. Sampling makes use of the Nyquist Frequency. According to the Nyquist Theorem, any signal must be sampled twice in order to reproduce it accurately. The formula is given by:

Nyquist Frequency = 1 / 2 (Dwell Time)

- **The dwell time in this formula refers to the time between two data points.**

When the frequency encoding gradient is turned on, the gradient has to be on long enough (sampling time) to receive and sample a range of frequencies bandwidth (receive bandwidth) in order to map it on the field of view (FOV) in the frequency direction. For example if there are 512 samples received, there must be at least 256 cycles that must occur during the sampled time if each cycle is to be sampled twice.

256 (cycles) x 2 (sampled times) = 512 samples

- Listed are two important rules to remember about sampling rate and sampling time.

1) **Sampling rate is proportional to receive bandwidth. If bandwidth increases, the sampling rate will also increase in order to get 2 cycles needed to represent it accurately.**

2) **Sampling time is inversely proportional to the sampling rate and the receive bandwidth. If the sampling rate and the receive bandwidth are reduced, the sampling time will have to be increase in order to get the 2 cycles needed to represent it accurately.**

K- Space

K- Space is the place where the signals, from the frequency axial and the phase axis, are collected until the scan is over. The images are then processed by the Fast Fourier Transform, mathematical process which makes the image. K-space is rectangular shape and has two axis, frequency and phase. The number of "rows" in K-space represents the number of phase encoding steps. The number of "columns", on the other hand, represents the number of data points the echo sampled. The direction of polarity for frequency travels right to left (negative) and travels left to right (positive) through K-space.

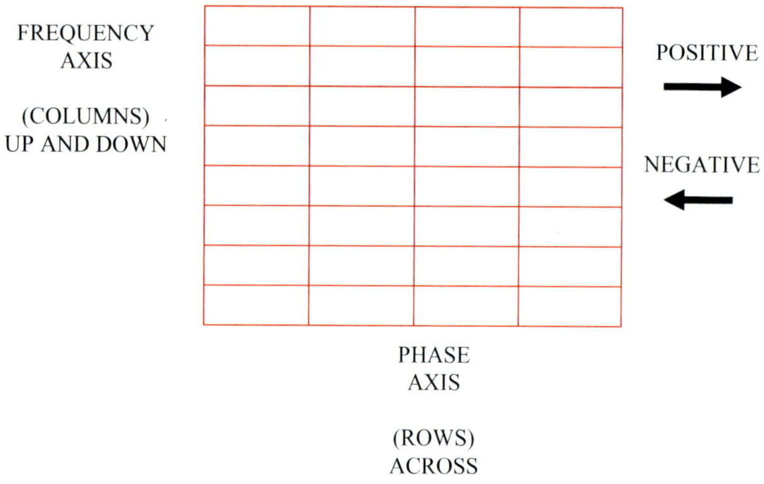

There are two types of filling of K-space, in which data can be obtained. The first way is called Sequential Filling. In this type of filling, the data is collected in a sequence of top to bottom. This means the phase encoding gradient positive fills the top half in the order of top to bottom. The phase encoding gradient negative fills the bottom half in the order of top to bottom.

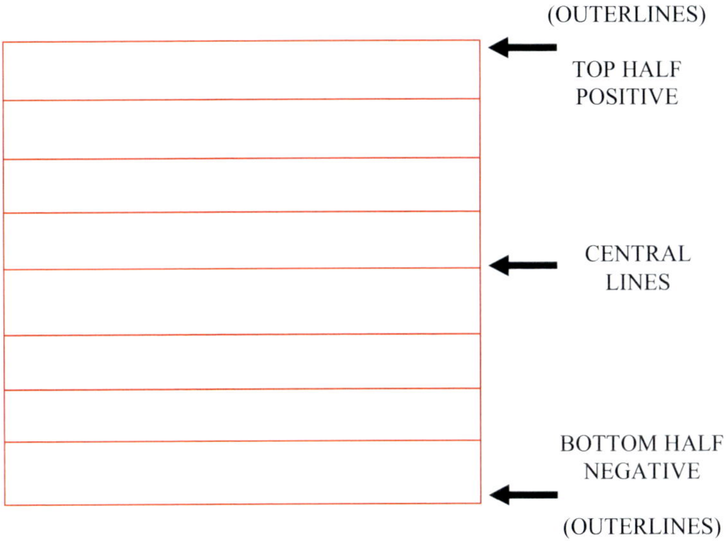

The second type of filling in K- space is called Centric Filling. In this type of filling, it starts at the center of K- space and works it way outward alternating between the positive and negative values.

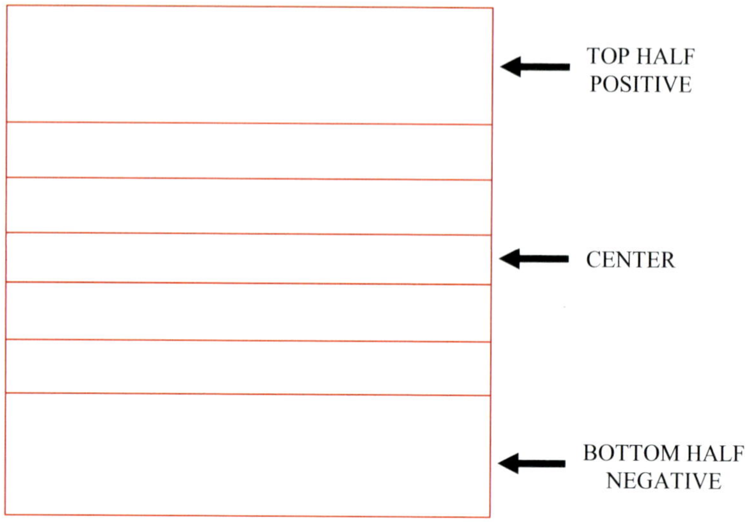

Another important concept deals with resolution. The outside of K- space contains the most resolution because it is filled by steep phase encoding gradients. The center lines of K- space have a low resolution because it is filled by shallow phase encoding gradients. The central part of K- space is good for signal to noise ratio (SNR) and contrast of the image.

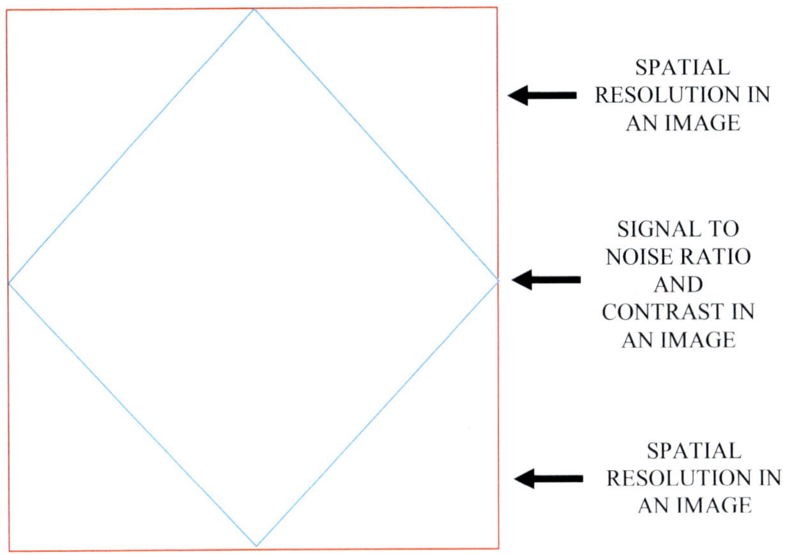

There are also two optional ways to collect K- space data besides sequential and centric. These are Partial or Fractional (Echo) Imaging and Partial or Fractional Averaging (Half Nexing). In fractional echo imaging, only part of the echo is collected. This is done to reduce the TE of the imaging sequence, which provides increase T1 weighting and PD weighting of an image. It also increases the number of slices that can be used for an image.

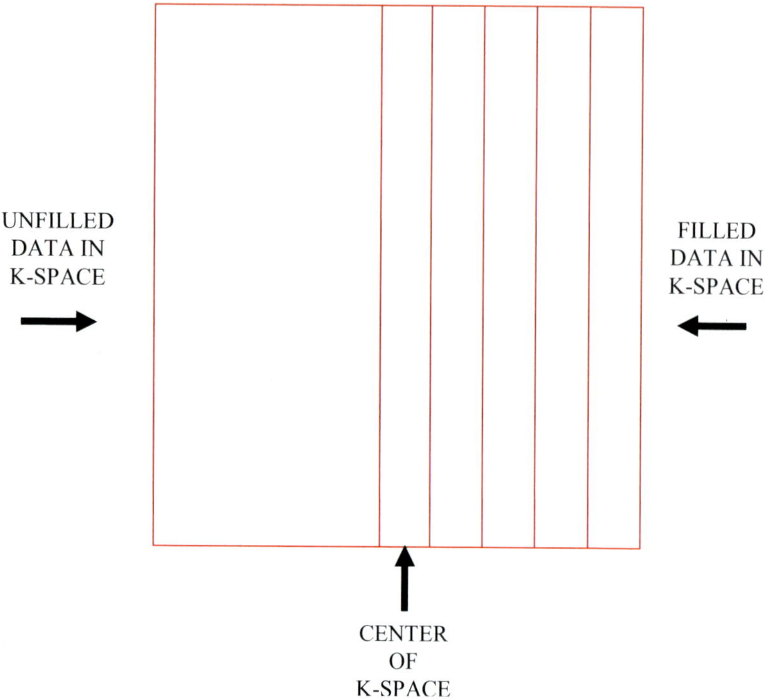

In partial or fractional averaging (half nexing), only part of the phase encoding steps are collected. The primary purpose of this is to reduce scan time.

FILLED
DATA IN
K-SPACE
CENTER OF
AXIS IN
K-SPACE
UNFILLED
DATA IN
K-SPACE

Chapter 5

Parameters and Trade – Offs

Parameter and trade – offs are two of the most important concepts in MRI when trying to obtain an optimal image. In MRI, it is usually a challenge to determine what parameters need to be adjusted. Although the philosophy of MRI scanning involves good signal to noise ratio, high resolution, and a short scan time, this concept does not always hold true. MRI utilizes the principle of give and take. If you change one parameter to acquire a good effect, something else will go lacking. For example, if you want good signal to noise ratio (SNR), the scan time may take longer than usual. This can lead to patient motion, which will affect resolution. In this chapter, some basic parameters and definitions are explained. The benefits and limitations of the basic parameters are also explained.

Spatial Resolution

Although this is a not a parameter on the MRI scanner, the concept of spatial resolution is important in terms of the other parameters. In spatial resolution, small means "clear" while large means "unclear". For example if an object is in a smaller perimeter, it will be clearer than if it is in a larger perimeter.

Scan Time

Scan time is the time of the actual scan. The formula is:

Scan Time = (TR) x (Number of phase encoding steps) x (NEX)

- The TR is the repetition time of the RF pulse.

- The number of phase encoding steps was explained in chapter four.

- The NEX is the number of times the phase encoding steps are sampled.

Scan time can increase by increasing TR, the number of phase encoding steps, or the NEX. Scan time can decrease by decreasing any of the three.

Slice Thickness

Slice thickness is the depth of the MRI slices. We learned in chapter four, slice thickness is chosen according to the anatomy being scanned. It deals with the concept of signal to noise ratio and spatial resolution of the image. If slice thickness increases, more anatomy will be covered, which increases signal to noise ratio. Spatial resolution decreases due to the excess noise accumulated by the scan, due to sampling. The opposite principle applies if slice thickness decreases.

Slice Gap or Spacing

This parameter deals with the space between slices. If spacing increases, there will be more distance covered, which increases signal to noise ratio. Spatial resolution decreases due to the excess noise accumulated by the scan, due to sampling.

Matrix

Matrix is the number of rows and columns of pixels in our image. For instance, if 256 pixels are in the columns section (frequency) and 128 pixels are in the rows section (phase), the matrix size would be 256 x 128. The parameters of matrix affects signal to noise ratio, spatial resolution, and scan time. If the matrix decreases, scan time and spatial resolution decreases while SNR increases.

COURSE OR
UNEVEN
MATRIX

256 X 128
FOR EXAMPLE

Scan time decreases because the number of phase encoding steps is reduced. Spatial resolution also decreases because the matrix is large, thus increasing signal to noise ratio. Due to increasing SNR, more noise accumulates, therefore degrading the scan. If the matrix size increases, spatial resolution and scan time increases while SNR decreases.

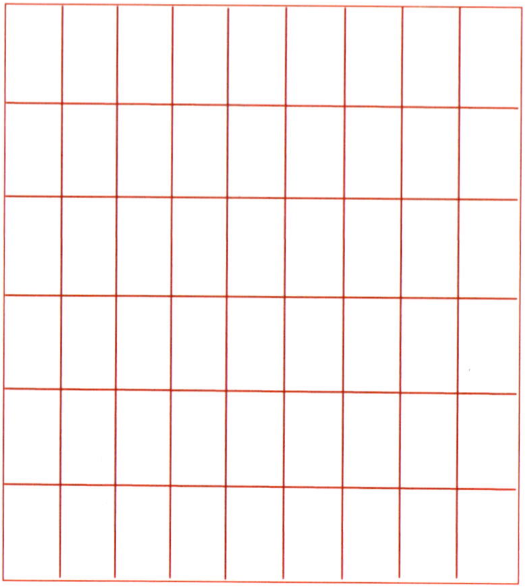

FINE OR
EVEN MATRIX

256 X 256
FOR EXAMPLE

Scan time increases because of the many phase encoding steps. Spatial resolution also increases due to the small matrix size. This allows less noise to accumulate by sampling in relation to signal collected.

Field of View

Field of view is the field of the scan. It is composed of the frequency encoding gradient and the phase encoding gradient. This parameter affects signal to noise ratio and spatial resolution. The same concept for the matrix applies for the

FOV. If the FOV increases, the SNR increases. This will cause spatial resolution to decrease, due to the increased noise sampled in addition to the signal. If the FOV decreases, the SNR decreases. This will cause spatial resolution to increase, due to the decreased noise sampled in addition to the signal.

- Listed is a diagram of the FOV and Spatial Resolution concept.

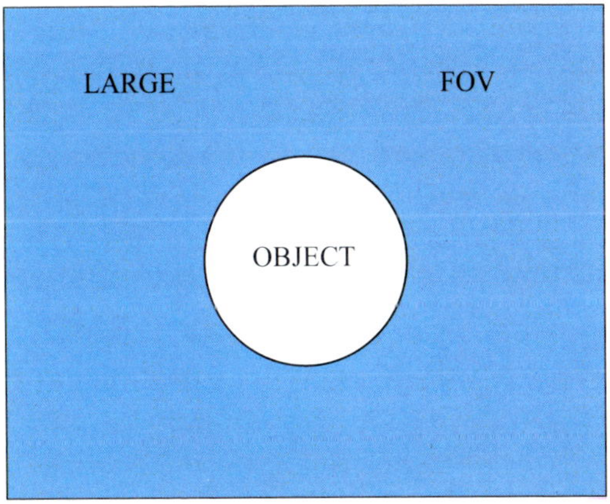

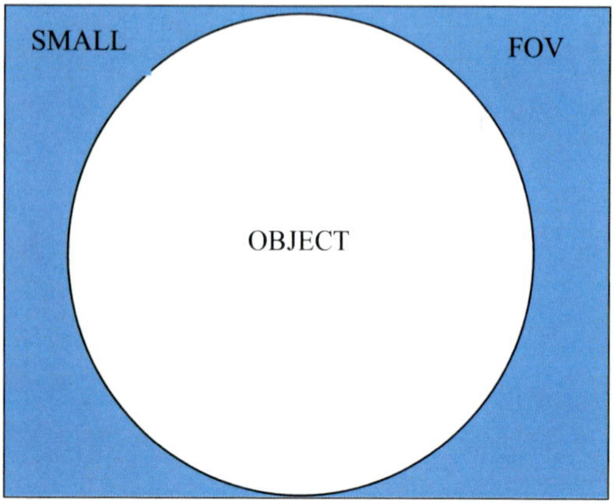

NEX (Number of Excitations)

NEX is defined as the number of times the phase encoding steps are sampled. Increasing sampling increases scan time and signal to noise ratio. For instance, if NEX increases from 2 to 4, the phase encoding steps are sampled 4 times instead of 2 times. Therefore, "if NEX doubles, scan time doubles also".

The disadvantage of NEX deals with SNR. Signal to noise ratio increases if NEX increases. This is defined as the square root of NEX or the square root of 2. In layman's terms, SNR increases by 41 % if NEX doubles. If NEX decreases, signal to noise ratio and scan time decreases due to less signal averaging.

Bandwidth

Bandwidth deals with SNR collected. If the bandwidth increases, more noise (41 %) will be collected. This reduces overall signal to noise ratio. If the bandwidth decreases, less noise will be collected. This improves signal to noise ratio.

- Listed is a diagram of the Receive Bandwidth and SNR concept.

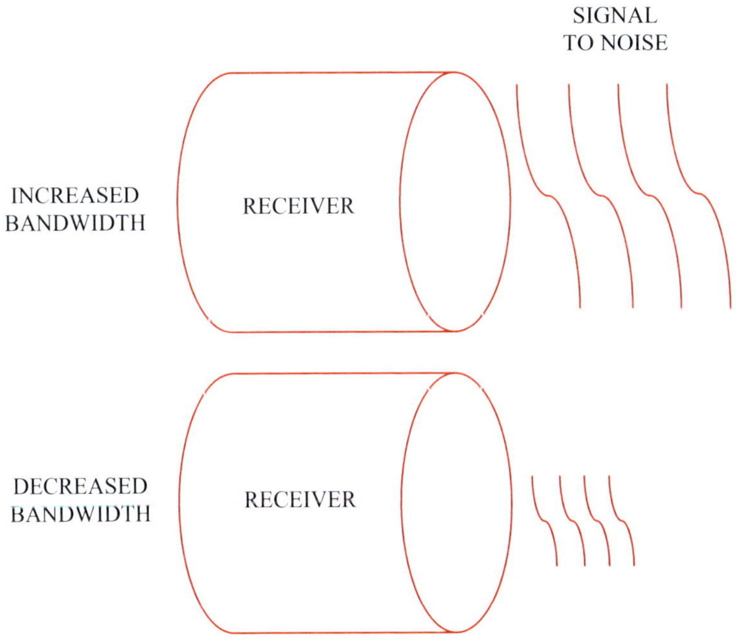

TR (Repetition Time)

Repetition time is the time when the RF pulse is applied to hydrogen or spins in our body. TR plays a major factor in scan time, the number of allowable slices, image weighting, and SNR.

In relation to scan time, increasing the repetition time increases scan time while decreasing the TR decreases scan time. The shorten scan time is used to reduce patient motion.

In relation to allowable slices, the MRI scanner can acquire more slices if TR increases. Decreasing the TR decreases the number of allowable slices. Image weighting is controlled by the repetition time as well.

In chapter two, we learned a short TR increases T1 and PD contrast weighted scans. A long TR increases T2 contrast weighted scans. Repetition time also plays a role in signal to noise ratio. Increasing the TR produces a high SNR. The scanner is allowed to be turn on, for a long period of time, in order to collect a high-quality signal from the spins. Decreasing the TR produces a low SNR. The scanner is not allowed to be turn on, for a long period of time, in order to collect a high-quality signal from the spins.

- Listed is a diagram of the TR and SNR concept.

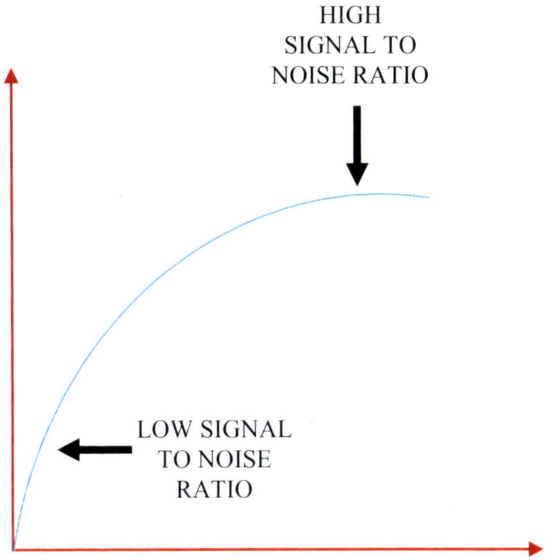

TE (Echo Time)

TE is the time it takes to sample the signal from the initial RF pulse to the collection of the echo. The echo time is an important factor in image weighting and signal to noise ratio. In chapter two, we learned a long TE time increases T2 contrast weighting in an image. A short TE time increases T1 contrast weighting in an image. The echo time also plays a role in SNR. Signal to noise ratio is higher as TE decreases. This occurs when the signal is sampled before the dcaying process begins. Signal to noise ratio is lower as TE time increases. This happens because the signal is sampled after the dcaying process has begun.

- Listed is a diagram of the TE and SNR concept.

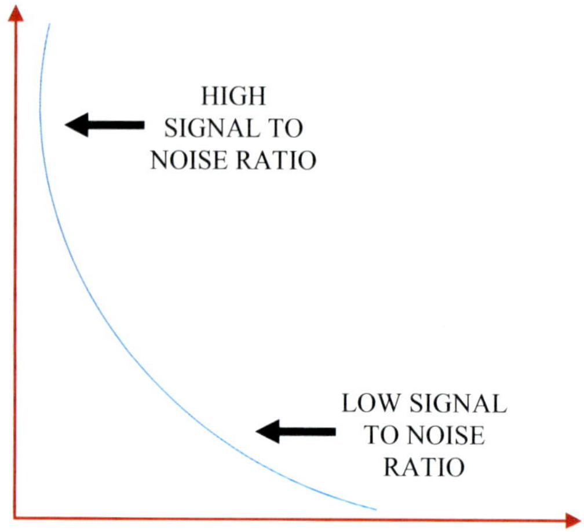

Flip Angle

In chapter one, we learned a flip angle is the RF pulse needed to move hydrogen or spins from the B_0 field to the B1 field (transverse plane). This parameter effects signal to noise ratio and contrast. Increasing the flip angle moves spins into the transverse plane, which increases SNR. The large flip angle influences T1 contrast weighting in an image. Decreasing the flip angle moves a small amount of spins into the transverse plane, which decreases SNR. The small flip angle influences T2* contrast weighting in an image.

- Listed is a diagram of the Flip Angle and SNR concept.

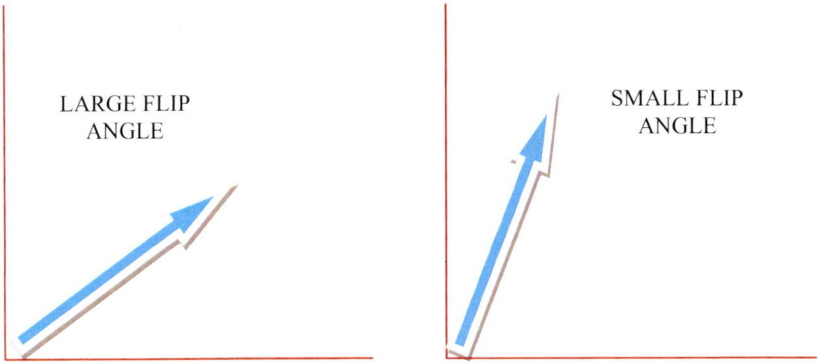

ETL (Echo Train Length), ETS (Echo Train Spacing), ETE (Effective Echo Time)

The ETL, ETS, and ETE are three parameters used in the Fast Spin Echo Sequence. The echo train length is the total number of signals collected during one TR period of a particular slice.

- Listed is a diagram that illustrates 1 TR period by showing the 90 degrees pulse and two 180 degrees pulse. There are 2 signals collected or 2 ETL.

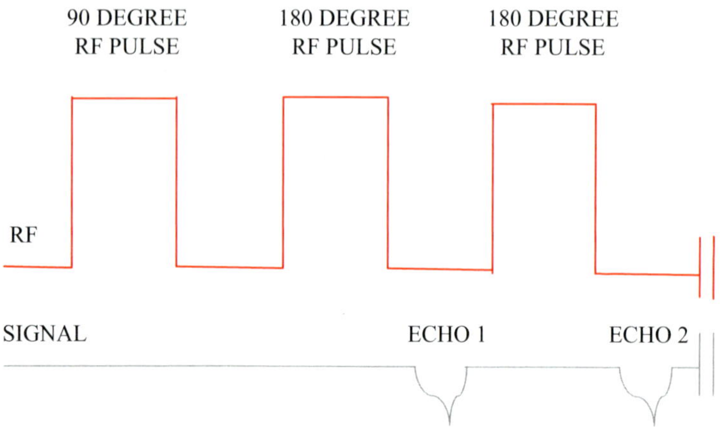

The ETL has a direct effect on scan time. The formula for a Fast Spin Echo is:

Scan Time = (TR) x (Number of phase encoding steps) x (NEX) / ETL

- **This means scan time increases if ETL decreases and vice versa. ETL also increases T2 contrast weighting if it increases. One bad effect of ETL is blurring, if the ETL increases to high.**

Echo Train Spacing (ETS)

ETS is the spacing between each echo in the multiple fast spin echo sequence. If more than one echo is present, each echo is totaled and divided by the number of echoes. The ETS, like the ETL, increases T2 weighting if it increases. The ETS also causes blurring if it increases to high.

- Listed is a diagram of Echo Train Spacing.

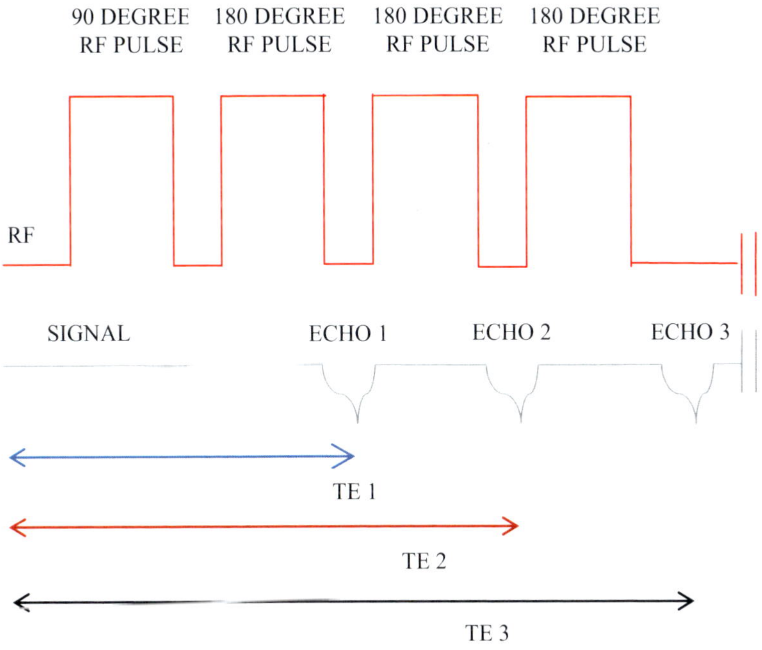

TE 1 = 30msec TE 2 = 50msec TE 3 = 70msec

ETS = 50msec

Effective Echo Time (ETE)

This parameter is similar to TE in spin echo sequences. ETE is the echo time needed to collect the signal when the phase encoding gradient is near zero (the center line of the phase encoding direction). This parameter also contributes the most to the contrast of the image, in a fast spin echo sequence. ETE, like the ETL and ETS, increases T2 weighting contrast if it increases. The ETE also decreases SNR if it decreases, as in spin echo sequences.

Chapter 6

Pulse Sequences

In this chapter, several common pulse sequences will be explained. As a MRI Technologist, it is extremely important to understand pulse sequences. Through these sequences, different gradients and parameters can be applied. Pulse sequences can be difficult to comprehend because they have good and bad effects on images. These good and bad effects will be explained in layman's terms, in order to make these concepts a little easier to understand.

Spin Echo (Conventional)

In chapter three, we learned a spin echo occurs when a 90 degrees RF pulse is applied to the B_0 field. This pulse will move the hydrogen spins to the B1 field. Once this happens, a 180 degrees pulse is applied to the hydrogen, which refocuses the spins. The signal or FID that comes from the refocusing echo is collected.

The spin echo sequence is often preferred to as the "Gold Standard" of MRI images because it provides the following: very good image quality, very versatile, and a true T2 weighting contrast that is sensitive to pathology.

In chapter two, we learned T1 weighting contrast is due to a short TR time and a short TE time. T2 weighting contrast is due to a long TR and a long TE time. Proton density weighting contrast is due to a long TR time and a short TE time. The spin echo sequence should be used whenever possible due to their excellent display of pathology and their high signal to noise ratio capabilities.

The only disadvantage of the spin echo sequence is scan times are very long. Long scan times are not optimal in MRI scanning. This can lead to patient motion.

- One way that helped me to understand the imaging sequences of spin echo, fast spin echo, and gradient echo are to think of them in terms of traveling on a trip. I compared the spin echo sequence to a bus trip. When you ride a bus to a certain destination, it takes longer to get there. By riding a bus, more of the scenery and details of the trip can be observed. This concept applies to the spin echo sequence. It may take longer to perform the scan, but the image spatial resolution is very good at the end of the scan.

- Listed is a diagram of the Spin Echo Sequence

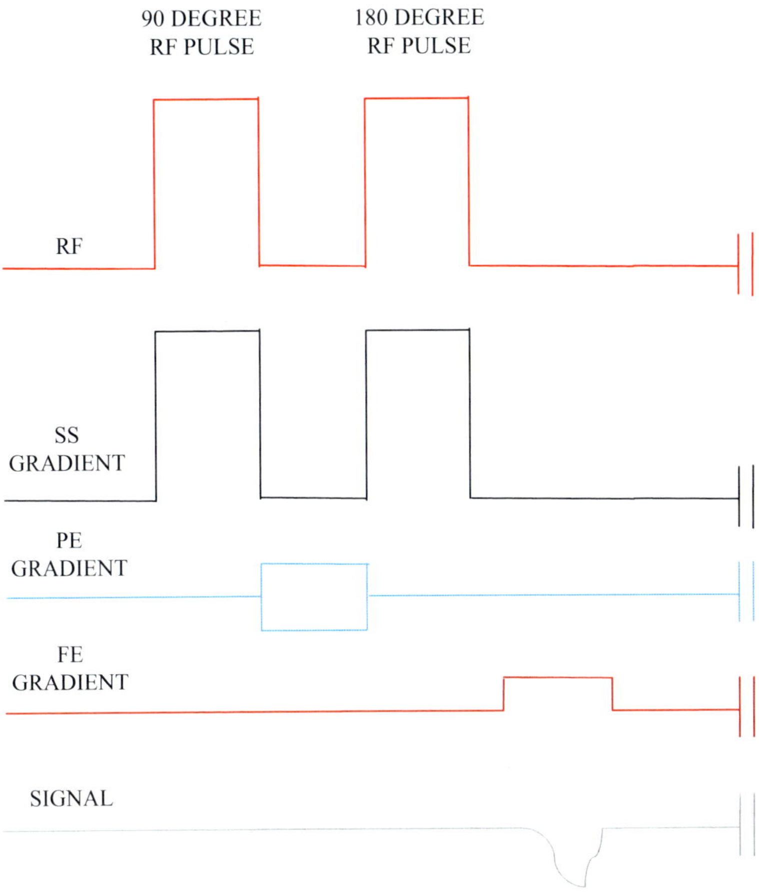

Fast Spin Echo (FSE)

The fast spin echo sequence is similar to the spin echo sequence. In a FSE, a 90 degrees RF pulse is applied to the spins; however, more than one 180 degrees RF pulse is applied to the spins. The numbers of 180 degrees RF pulses determine the number of echoes produced and the number of K- space lines that are filled.

We learned in chapter five, the FSE uses the parameter ETL, ETS, and ETE. We also learned a T1 weighed contrast image is causes by a short TR time, a short TE time, and an ETL of 2- 6. Proton Density contrast weighting is due to a long TR time, a short TE time, and an ETL of 8-12. T2 weighting is due to a long TR time, a long TE time, and an ETL of 12- 20.

The fast spin echo sequence provides relatively good image quality; high spatial resolution matrices, multiple NEX that can be used, excellent T2 weighted contrast image, and scan times are greatly reduced.

Some of the disadvantages of a FSE includes: increased blurring of the image (due to collecting data at different TE's) and increased flow and motion artifacts. Hemorrhages (blood pools), a disadvantage, should not be examined with this scan, due to the reduced magnetic susceptibility effects. Fatty substances also appear bright or hyperintense on T2 weighted contrast images. All of these disadvantages are due to the mixing of the echo times.

- Referring back to the last section about imaging sequences (SE, FSE, and GE) and traveling on a trip, the fast spin echo sequence can be compared to a train trip. The train goes a little faster than the bus; however, only some of the scenery and details can be seen along the way. This concept applies to the fast spin echo sequence. FSE reduces scan time, compared to a spin echo, and the spatial resolution is relatively good at the end of the scan.

- Listed is a diagram of the Fast Spin Echo Sequence

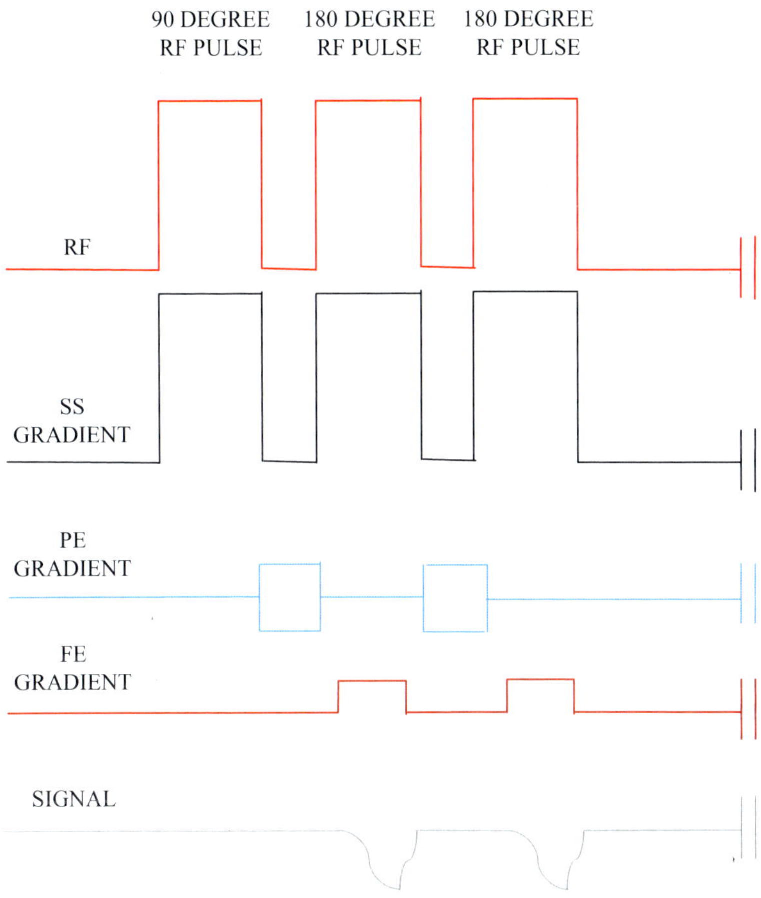

Inversion Recovery (IR)

The Inversion Recovery sequence involves suppression of certain tissues within the image. It begins with the application of a 180 degrees RF pulse, which inverts the net magnetization vector into full saturation. Once the RF pulse is turned off, the vector will try to relax back to equilibrium or B_o. While the vector is relaxing back, a 90 degrees excitation pulse called TI (inversion time) is applied to the vector. The formula for suppression is:

Suppression = .69 x (T1 of tissue that is being suppressed by IR)

In the IR sequence, the contrast depends on the length of the TI or inversion time. The TR time, in this sequence, will always be long in comparison to the other imaging scans. The scan needs to be on long enough to allow suppression to take place. For a T1 weighted contrast image, the TR time is long (2000msec and above), the TE time is short (10 – 20msec), and the TI time is medium (400 – 800msec). In a PD contrast weighted image, the TR time is long (2000msec and above), the TE time is short (10 –20msec), and the TI time is long (1800msec). For a pathology contrast weighted image, the TR time is long (2000msec and above), the TE time is long (70msec and above), and the TI time is medium (400 – 800msec).

Some advantages of the inversion recovery sequence includes: a very high SNR (due to the long TR time) and enhanced discrimination between tissues with close T1's. It creates heavily T1 contrast weighted images and also be used for signal suppression.

The disadvantages are increase power to the patient (due to the additional 180 degrees RF pulse) and long scan times (due to the additional TI time in the sequence). The IR sequence is mainly used for PD and T1 contrast weighted imaging. It will not produce a signal if the TI time is not chosen properly. It is usually best to use an IR sequence in conjunction with a FSE sequence in order to reduce long scan times.

There are two common types of inversion recovery sequences: STIR and FLAIR. STIR (Short TI Inversion Recovery Sequence) is an IR sequence used to suppress fatty substances on MRI images. The parameters used for this sequence are a long TR time (2000msec and above), a short TE time (10 – 20msec), and a short TI time (150 – 175msec).

FLAIR (Fluid Attenuated Inversion Recovery) is an IR sequence used to suppress fluid filled substances, like CSF, on MRI images. The parameters used for this sequence are a long TR time (6000msec and above), a short or long TE time (depending on contrast weighting required for the image), and a long TI time (1700 – 2200msec).

- Listed is a diagram of the typical Inversion Recovery Sequence

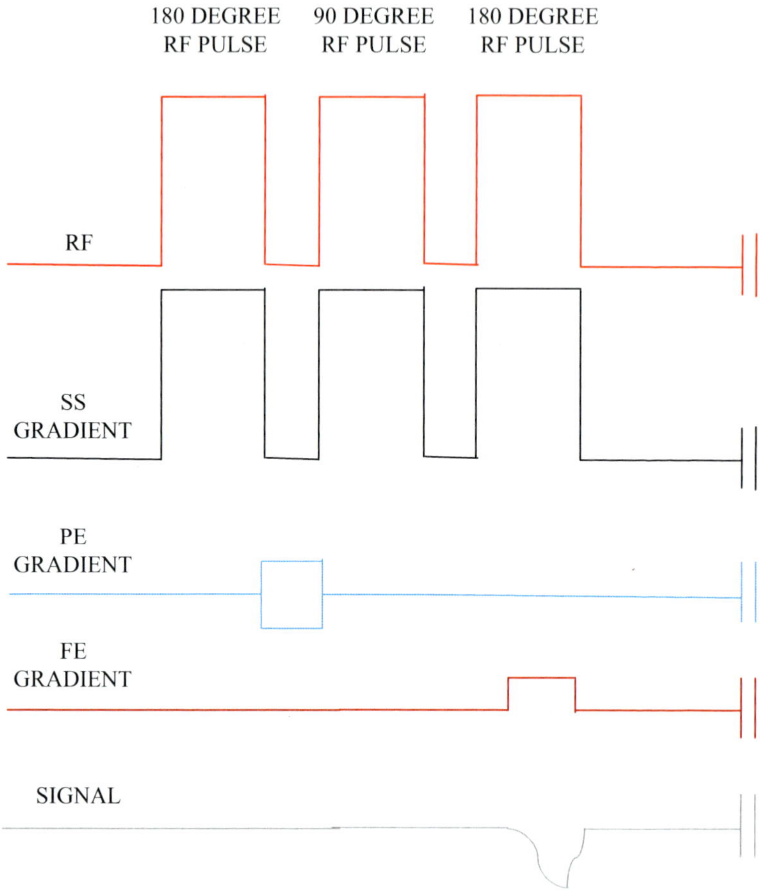

Gradient Echo (GE)

We learned in chapter three, a gradient echo occurs when an RF excitation pulse is applied to the B_o field. This pulse will move the hydrogen spins to the B1 field. Once this happens, a gradient reversal is used to refocus the spins. The signal or FID which comes from the refocusing echo is collected.

The gradient echo sequence is a very fast scan due to a short TR time. It also reduces power deposition to the patient. The only disadvantage of the gradient echo sequence is it suffers from T2* relaxation. This means T2* effects, which are caused by magnet inhomogeneities, magnet susceptibility inhomogeneities and chemical shifts dispersion (different larmar frequencies) will not be refocused. This causes a loss of MRI signal.

We also learned in chapter two, the parameters related to contrast weighting in conventional GE sequences. For a T1 contrast weighted image, the TR time is short (less than 50msec), the TE time is short (5 – 10msec), and the flip angle is large (70 – 100 degrees). For a T2* contrast weighted image, the TR time is short (less than 50msec), the TE time is long (15 – 25msec), and the flip angle is small (5 – 70 degrees). For a PD contrast weighted image, the TR time is short (less than 50msec), the TE time is short (5 – 10msec), and the flip angle is small (5 – 70 degrees).

- Referring back to the section about imaging sequences (SE, FSE, GE) and traveling on a trip, the GE sequence can be compared to a plane. A plane arrives at a destination quickly; however, the scenery and details of the trip will not be clear. This concept applies to the gradient echo sequence. The scan is extremely fast, on the other hand, the spatial resolution is not very good at the end of the scan. This is due to the speed of the scan and the loss of signal from T2* effects.

- Listed is a diagram of the typical Gradient Spin Echo

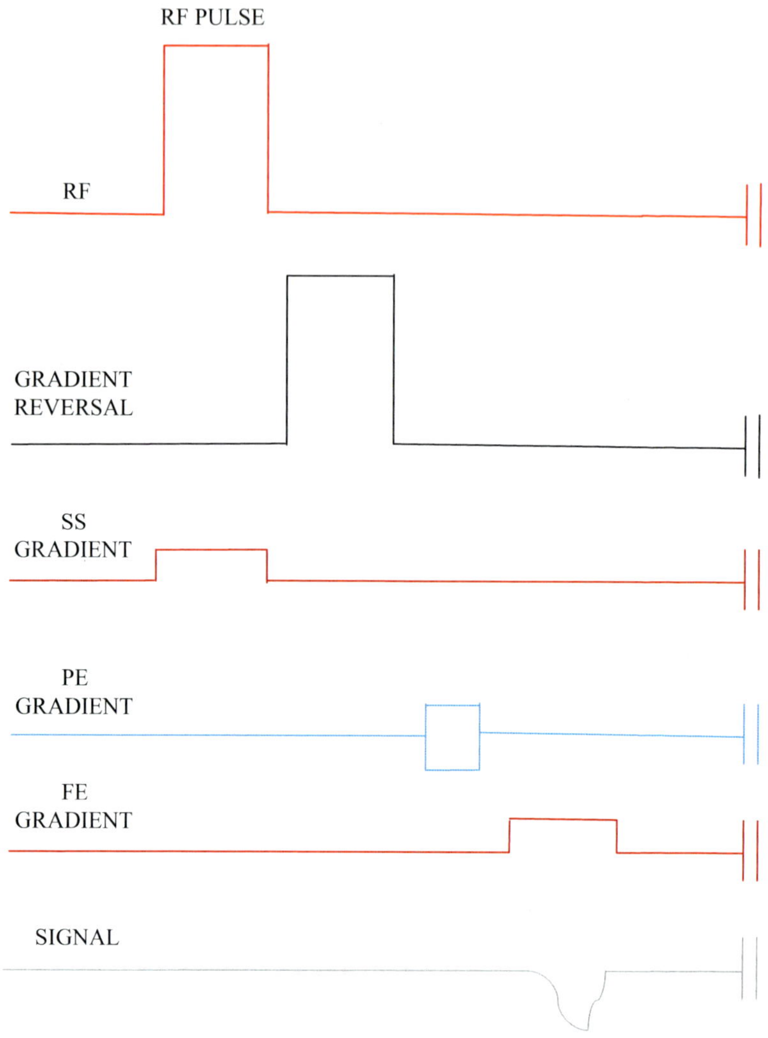

Steady State Gradient Echo Sequence

Before we go any further, let's discuss the principle of the steady state of gradient echo sequences. It is important to understand this concept prior to learning about the three common types of gradient echo sequences (Coherent, Incoherent, and Steady State Free Precession).

So what is a steady state? The steady state occurs when the TR time is chosen so short, the T1 (rephrasing) or T2* (dephasing) relaxation will not take effect. In layman's terms, the addition of RF pulse will set up a steady state, of the spins, after they are hit by the TR many times.

The steady state gradient echo sequence collects two signals. One is collected for incomplete T1 relaxation and the other one for incomplete T2* relaxation. The echo collected from the incomplete T1 is called the FID. The echo collected from the T2* relaxation is called the residual (dephasing portion of the spin echo) transverse magnetization. This is called stimulated echoes or Hahm spin echo. It will affect contrast by allowing tissues with long T2* times to appear bright on the scan or image.

Coherent Steady State

The coherent steady state gradient sequence is similar to conventional gradient echo sequences. A variable RF excitation flip angle or pulse is applied to the B_0 field. This pulse will move the hydrogen spins to the B1 field. Once this happens, a phase encoding gradient reversal produces the signal.

In the coherent sequence, gradients called "rewinders" are applied after the phase encoding gradient. These gradients will reverse or rewind the spins of the phase encoding gradient after the readout gradient collects signals from the spins. This rephrasing, of the FID and the Hahn echo, allows the residual magnetization to build up so tissues with long T2 times will produce a bright signal.

The coherent steady state scan is mainly used to produce T2* contrast weighting in gradient echo sequences. This scan is very fast (allowing breath hold exams), gives good angiography studies (show vessels bright), and is used for 3D volumetric imaging.

The disadvantage of the scan is it produces poor SNR and is very loud due to the present of the steady state. The scan also increases T2* relaxation due to magnetic susceptibilities.

The parameters used in this sequence involves a flip angle (30 – 45 degrees), a short TR time (20 – 50msec), and a long TE time (15 – 25msec) to maximize T2* contrast weighting. In order to decrease T2* contrast weighting, the shortest possible TE time should be used. This allows T1 and PD contrast weighting on the images.

Incoherent Residual Transverse Magnetization

The incoherent or spoiled residual transverse magnetization is similar to conventional gradient echo sequences. A variable RF excitation flip angle or pulse is applied to the B_o field. This pulse will move the hydrogen spins to the B1 field. Once this happens, gradient rephasing is used to produce the signal.

In the incoherent sequence, gradients are used to rephase the FID only and not the hahm echo. In this sequence, the hahm echo is spoiled by Gradient Spoiling or by Digitized RF

Spoiling. The concept of gradient spoiling is opposite of rewinding in the coherent sequence. In the coherent sequence, the residual magnetization is allowed to build up in tissues with long T2 times by rephrasing the hahm echo. In the incoherent sequence, the residual magnetization is not allowed to build up. The residual magnetization is dephased by the slice selection, phase encoding, and readout gradients. This dephasing will reduce T2* effects, while increasing T1 and PD effects. The hahm echo can also be spoiled by RF spoiling (this is more efficient than gradient spoiling). In RF spoiling, the receiver coil which collects the signals will lock on to a specific phase of the RF pulse that is transmitted. Only signals from that RF pulse will be collected while the other signals, not locked on, will be spoiled.

The incoherent scan is mainly used to produce T1 and PD weighting in gradient echo sequences. This scan is very fast (allowing breath hold exams) and is used for 2D or 3D exams.

The disadvantage of the scan is it produces poor SNR, due to the present of the steady state.

The parameters used in this sequence involves a flip angle (30 – 45 degrees), a short TR time (20 – 50msec), and a short TE time (5 – 10msec) to maximize T1 contrast weighting on the image.

Steady State Free Precession (SSFP)

We learned earlier in this chapter, the steady state sequence is a very fast scan. The steady state sequence uses the shortest possible TR time, in order to perform this scan. Due to this circumstance, the TE time is never long enough to give a true measure of T2 contrast weighting. So the steady state free precession sequence was created. The steady state free precession sequence uses a series of RF pulse to start the echo. The SSFP sequence is also involved in the rephrasing process of the scan. This sequence uses rewinder gradients; however, the rewinder in the steady state free precession sequence is used to reposition the signal to a time when it can be collected. It only collects the signal of the hahm echo.

This scan is mainly used to get a true T2 contrast weighted image in gradient echo sequences. It is also used for 2D or 3D exams.

The disadvantage of this scan is it produces poor SNR and is very loud due to the present of the steady state. This scan is also susceptible to artifacts.

The parameters used in this sequence involve a flip angle (30 – 45 degrees), a short time (20 – 50msec), and a short time (5 – 10msec) to maximize T1 effects. This sequence also involves an actual TE time and an effective TE time. The actual TE time, in this sequence, affects the effective TE time in the image. This means decreasing the TE time will actually increase the effective TE time seen in the image unless a fixed TE time is used.

Chapter 7

Flow Phenomena and Compensation

As a student, the concept of flow phenomena was difficult to comprehend. The issue of "flowing" involves nuclei that exhibit different contrast characteristics from neighboring stationary nuclei. The movement of flowing nuclei will lead to mismapping of the signals and results in artifacts called flow motion artifacts or phase ghosting. In this chapter, flow phenomena and compensation will be explained. By putting these concepts in layman's terms, the principles of flow phenomena and compensation can be better understood.

Types of Flow

Before we learn about the principles behind flow phenomena, let's discuss the five type of flow. There are five types of flow: Plug flow, Laminar flow, Turbulent flow, Vortex flow, and Stagnant flow.

Plug flow occurs when the flow has a constant velocity across the vessel. Laminar flow occurs when flow, in the center of the vessel, is faster than flow at the vessel wall. This is due to the resistance at the wall slowing down the vessel flow. Turbulent flow occurs when flow travels at different velocities in the vessels. This flow fluctuates randomly and is erratic. Vortex flow starts out as laminar flow but then it passes through a stricture in the vessel. Once the flow passes through the stricture, it becomes erratic and "re- circulation" zones can occur. Stagnant flow is flow that moves very low.

Flow mechanisms are often termed as:

- **1st order motion which is laminar flow**
- **2nd order motion which is accelerated motion**
- **3rd order motion which is jerk motion**

- At the present time, only 1st order flow can be compensated for.

Time of Flight (TOF)

We learned in chapter six, to produce a signal, the nuclei or a nucleus must receive an excitation pulse and a rephasing pulse or gradient reversal. If a nucleus receives an excitation pulse and is not rephased, then a MRI signal will not be produced. In order to produce a MRI signal, the nuclei must be excited and rephased. If this does not occur, the moving nuclei will result in a signal void (dark appearance) in spin echo sequences or flow related enhancement (bright appearance) in gradient echo sequences. This is the philosophy of the time of fight phenomena.

In spin echo sequences, TOF effects increase as velocity and TE times increase. For example, if the spins move very fast or have long TE times, they will move outside of the slices before they are rephased. On the other hand, TOF effects decrease with a thicker slice rather than with a thinner slice.

In a thicker slice, the spins can be rephased before they leave the slice. In a thinner slice; however, TOF increases because the spins do not have time to be rephased before they leave the slice.

In gradient echo sequences, TOF effects are the exact opposite of spin echo sequences. Flow related enhancement increases with decrease (slower) velocity of flow and with decrease (shorter) TE times. In gradient echo sequences, the excitation pulse is a slice selective pulse. However, the rephasing gradient is non selective and is applied to the whole body. Due to the slow movement of the spins or the TE time being short, the spins can be excited and rephased by the rephasing gradient since this gradient is applied to the entire body. Flow related enhancement also increases with a thicker slice rather than with a thinner slice. If the slice is thick, for example, the spin has a better chance of being excited and rephased in comparison to a thinner slice.

Entry Slice Phenomena (IN Flow Effects)

The principles of entry slice phenomena or in flow effects can be tough to understand. These principles will be explained in layman's terms. Entry slice phenomena deal with the ability of the stationary nuclei or spins to become saturated. This is done by the application of applying repeated RF pulses to the nuclei. If the nuclei are not saturated, it will appear bright in gradient echo sequences. An entry slice phenomenon is usually seen in the first slice of an imaging series because the nuclei have not become saturated. However, if these effects are seen in slice 2 through infinity then there is a concern.

When it comes to the principle of in flow effects, it is wise to think of a stack of slices in a row (for example 1 – 10). A decrease (short) TR time, a decrease (slower) velocity of flow, and an increase (thick) in slice thickness will decrease entry slice effects. If the TR time is short, more RF pulses will be applied to the spins at a higher rate. If the velocity of the spins is slower than normal, the spins can easily become saturate by the RF pulses. If the slice thickness is thick rather than thin, the spins will not be able to move in and out of the slice before they are saturated.

The direction of flow also plays a factor in determining the entry slice phenomena. Co-current flow decreases in flow effects while counter-current increase it. In co-current flow, the spin goes in numerical order down the row of slices (1-10). If the spins travel in order, the RF pulses can catch up with the spins and saturate them. In counter-current flow, on the other hand, the spins do not travel in numerical order. They travel in descending numerical order in the row of slices (10-1). This will increase entry slice phenomena because the spins can't be saturated until later in the slice.

Summary of TOF and Entry Slice Phenomena

Increase Signal Voids	Increase Flow Enhancement
Increase Velocity (Fast)	Decrease Velocity (slow)
Increase TE (long)	Decrease TE (short)
Decrease Slice Thickness	Increase Slice Thickness

Increase In Flow Effects	Decrease In Flow Effects
At the first slice	At the first slice
Increase TR (Long)	Decrease TR (Short)
Decrease Slices (Thin)	Increase Slices (Thick)
Increase Flow (Fast)	Decrease Flow (Slow)
Counter-Current Flow	Co-Current Flow

Intra -Voxel Dephasing Phenomena

In chapter four, we learned the presence of a gradient gives a hydrogen spin or nuclei a specific value at a certain place inside of the magnet. We also learned gradients alter the static magnetic field. These two principles are the basis for the intra – voxel dephasing phenomena.

In the phenomena, there are nuclei flowing along a gradient at different accelerating rates (fast or slow). This process depends on the direction of flow and the direction of the gradient application. The fast moving nuclei are called gain phase. The slow moving nuclei are called lose phase. When these following nuclei meet in passing and are adjacent to the stationary nucleus in a voxel, there will be a difference in phase between the nuclei because of the motion along the gradient. This results in a loss of signal, from the voxel, called intra – voxel dephasing. If these effects occur in turbulent or vortex flow, the effects are irreversible. If intra – voxel dephasing occurs in laminar flow, the effects can be compensated for if the velocity of flow is constant.

Gradient Moment Nulling (Rephasing)

Gradient moment nulling is a method which uses additional gradients to compensate for the altered phase values (precessional frequencies) of nuclei flowing along the gradient. It does this by dephasing the flowing and stationary spins with the slice selection gradient or the readout gradient. This allows the flowing and stationary spins to have the same precessing frequencies, of nuclei, at the beginning and the end of the gradient application. Once this process occurs, all of the spins are in phase, thus reducing intra – voxel dephasing.

Gradient moment nulling is often called the first order of motion compensation because it is most effective on slow laminar flow rather than turbulent or vortex flow. Gradient moment nulling is usually used in T2 and T2* contrast weighted sequences because the flowing nuclei in these sequences are already bright. This is due to the flowing nuclei and the stationary spins having the same phase, thus producing a bright signal.

The disadvantage of gradient moment nulling is minimum TE increases, which decreases T1 and PD contrast weighted images. This is due to the extra gradient used. This sequence also decreases the number of slices which can be used in the scan.

Pre – saturation (SAT Band)

The concept behind the pre – saturation pulse or saturation (SAT) band is easy to comprehend. It involves applying a pre – saturation pulse (90 degrees) between the flow and the imaging stack so flowing blood coming into the FOV are nullified or voided. The SAT band can also be applied above and below the FOV to get rid of arterial and venous flow. Pre – saturation pulse are mainly used in T1 contrast weighted images, in order to minimize entry slice phenomena and TOF effects. They are also used for fat and water saturation and reduce aliasing artifacts.

The disadvantage of using a SAT band is it increases RF power deposition to the patient, due to the additional 90 degree RF pulse, and may decrease the number of slices used in the scan.

- In my opinion, a pre – saturation pulse is similar to the lead blocker on the x – ray tube. When performing x – rays, the lead blocker is put along side of the anatomy. These decreases scatter radiation and make the resolution of the image better. The same principle applies to the pre – saturation pulse. By applying the SAT band to the MRI image, it will nullify the flowing nuclei, thus making the resolution of the scan better.

Even Echo Rephasing

The principle of even echo rephasing is easy to comprehend. Earlier we learned, a fast spin echo sequence involves multiple echoes. Sometimes these echoes become out of phase (dephase) at the first echo time and will not become in phase (rephase) until the second echo time. This leads to intra – voxel dephasing. A way to reduce the intra – voxel dephasing is by using even echo rephasing. This process involves acquiring the second and succeeding even echoes at a multiple of the first TE. By collecting the even echoes, nuclei will have enough time to rephase themselves thus reducing artifacts in a T2 contrast weighted image. Even echo rephasing will only work if nuclei are given the exact amount of time to rephase as they were given to dephase.